YOGA FOR BEGINNERS

YOGA FOR BEGINNERS

A Simple Guide to the Best Yoga Styles and Exercises for Relaxation, Stretching, and Good Health

NTATHU ALLEN

Copyright © 2017 by Ntathu Allen

All Rights Reserved.

No part of this book may be reproduced, stored in retrieval systems, or transmitted by any means, electronic, mechanical, photocopying, recorded or otherwise without written permission from the author.

ISBN: 978-1-63161-043-1

Published by TCK Publishing

www.TCKPublishing.com

Get discounts and special deals on our best selling books at

www.tckpublishing.com/bookdeals

Illustrated by

Jamie Whipham

Disclaimer/Limitations of Liability

Some material in this book may have previously existed as blog posts or articles written by the author.

The aim of this book is to provide general information only and should not be treated as a substitute for the medical advice of your doctor or any other healthcare professional. The information is intended to help you choose the right style of yoga class for you. It is based on my personal and professional experience of studying and teaching yoga.

This book makes no guarantees of success or implied promises. The publisher and author are not responsible or liable for any diagnosis made by a reader based on the contents of this book. Always consult your doctor before starting the exercises in this book or if you are concerned about your health in any way.

Remember, as you practice the yoga and meditation exercises in this book, breathe in and out gently through your nose. Keep your awareness on your breathing, allow the movement to be gentle and loving, and stay attentive to what is happening inside your body. Thank you.

FOREWORD

THIS BOOK IS a treasure trove full of wisdom for all women. Immediately after I started reading, I felt inspired to start the practices Ntathu so easily introduces us to. The guidelines are easy to follow, and I instantly felt calm and relaxed with her easy-to-follow instructions.

Forget Yoga mats and Yoga classes and all the effort it takes to get out the door and to classes. At last, here's a workable book for the masses that brings yoga to your desk and to your home in a language and showing exercises, we can all understand.

In our time-poor, demanding work schedule and life culture, this book is a diamond. Using accessible language, Ntathu skillfully transforms the riches of yoga and transforms it into lay activities even a beginner can practice at work or at home.

I love the easy-to-follow chapters and bite-size yoga exercises, which have clearly been written by a seasoned/expert yoga practitioner who understands the plight of the working woman who doesn't have the time or even the will to attend the weekly yoga classes.

This is one book every woman—and man—should have a copy of. I plan to send copies to all my coaching clients as Christmas gifts. At last, we have an e-book that touches the part other books don't reach!

~Jackee Holder

Management and Leadership Coach, Author, and Speaker

www.jackeeholder.com

CONTENTS

Foreword v

Introduction ix

Chapter 1 Helpless to Hopeful on the Road to Recovery 1

Chapter 2 Stress to Success 9

Chapter 3 Crazy-Busy to Blissfully Calm 41

Chapter 4 Panic to Peace 59

Chapter 5 Final Thoughts for a Calmer, Happier You 67

Glossary of the Key Yoga Terms Used in This Book 69

About The Author 71

Index 80

INTRODUCTION

ARE YOU TIRED of being tired and grumpy, running on empty, giving everything to everyone at work and at home, and having nothing left for *you*?

Do you want to feel fitter, healthier, worry less, and have more energy, so you can have more fun and enjoy life?

Maybe you feel frazzled, frustrated, and fed-up at work yet suffer in silence.

Did you know that stress is recognized as the number one killer today? 62% of Americans are stressed about work, and one out of four working women admit to having taken a "mental-health day" because of work-related pressures.

If you feel as if your life is spinning out of control and no matter what you do, everything still weighs you down, then this book is for you.

Whether you are a stressed-out professional tired of living life in the fast-worry lane, or a busy parent who's exhausted from getting your children ready for school then dashing off to work, then take heart. *Yoga for Beginners: A Simple Guide to the Best Yoga Styles and*

Exercises for Relaxation, Stretching, and Good Health offers you inspiration, relaxation tips, and exercises to put your life back into balance.

All the yoga exercises, breathing exercises and meditation techniques can be safely done at home or at work. They are practices which I use and share with my yoga students.

This practical guide includes information on the dangers of stress and the benefits of yoga to enable you to feel better; easy–to-follow yoga exercises you can do at your work-station to de-stress; simple, deep-breathing exercises and meditation techniques to calm and revitalise your body; so you can quickly "switch off" from work mode and enjoy a peaceful evening at home.

As a yoga teacher, I am often asked by my students what they can do to regain that "post-yogic glow," especially at work when the pressure is on. At the end of their yoga lesson, students always sigh and state, "If only I could feel this good at work."

That's why I wrote this book.

My students needed take-away yoga to do at work and at home.

Mary, a 58-year-old accountant and a complete beginner at yoga says, "I have never felt so relaxed and free of pain." And after her first lesson, Cynthia, a yoga student with mental health issues, said, "My body feels really relaxed and stretched; I found the class to be more useful than I thought it would be."

If you would like to experience calm, feel relaxed, and become pain free, then this book is for you.

So, stop beating up on yourself. Sit back, take a deep breath, lower your shoulders, and enjoy easy living the yogic way.

1

HELPLESS TO HOPEFUL ON THE ROAD TO RECOVERY

Get Ready to Enjoy Your Stress-Free Life

DOES YOUR LIFE feel like a juggling act?

Do you feel torn between caring for your family and giving your full attention to your work?

Have you taken work home to complete or left work early to see your son perform in his school play and then felt guilty for doing either one of these things?

In this chapter, you will discover the frightening effects stress has on your life. You will find out what you can do to protect your body from physically breaking down and what you must do to stop your mind from running on overdrive with all the strain placed on you.

Reduce the Signs and Symptoms of Stress

Would you like to be calmer and more focused at work? To have energy to get through your day without "crashing out" in the afternoon and feeling drained when you leave work?

To feel healthier, happier and more at peace?

Can you imagine how happier you will feel if you could improve your health, have energy to walk up the stairs without puffing and not worry whether you are able to bend down and pick things up from the floor?

These are just some of the benefits you will discover as you explore the vast potential of yoga to release tension, stress and anxiety.

Too Many Demands on You?

How do you manage when your boss is asking questions about the overdue report and when you get home, your daughter reminds you, "You promised, Mum," to help her bake cakes for the school Sports Day? Do you bake the cakes and stay up late to finish your report then collapse into bed? Maybe you moan at your partner for not pulling his weight around the house.

Whilst doing all of this, where do you find time for you? You might desire to live a simpler life, to work fewer hours, or even change jobs and retrain to follow your childhood dreams. However, with the increased cost of living, higher medical bills, and the real threat of getting laid off, you fear taking time off.

> **Stress-free Fact:**
> Recent information states that 80% of all chronic illness is brought on by stress. It also has been shown that genetic-related illnesses are very frequently stress-related.

Do You Know the Toll Your Overworked Life Is Taking on You?

Constant overworking and lack of rest affects your physical, emotional, and spiritual health. When was the last time you cooked an evening meal and ate it with your family—undisturbed by the television, computer, phone calls or text messages?

This steady pressure and sense of rush pervades all aspects of a person's life, and if left unchecked, leads to anxiety, depression, stress-related disorders, and even alcoholism and drug dependency.

Signs and Symptoms of Workplace Stress

You spend a large proportion of your time at work. Therefore, being comfortable helps you to be more productive. Your inability to relax leads you to feel overworked, harassed, and undervalued. These feelings have a huge impact on the way you communicate with your bosses, colleagues, and clients. When you are discontented at work, your health suffers. This has a negative influence on your company's public profile, as it affects your ability to do your work properly.

The word stress means different things to different people.

Simply put, stress is reacting negatively to perceived unpleasant things in your life.

People use the word "stress" to describe how they feel when they struggle to cope with all the demands placed upon them. Learning to let go and to manage pressure empowers you to unwind and to have a more pleasurable and relaxed lifestyle.

Did You Know That Stress Is Recognized as the Number One Killer Today?

The American Medical Association states that stress is the cause of 80 to 85% percent of all human illness and disease.

Furthermore, every week, 95 million Americans suffer stress-related symptoms for which they take medication and, more than 22 billion dollars are spent on anxiety-related healthcare services each year.

Figures like that freak me out. Would you like to feel better, happier, less stressed out, more in control of your workload?

Or do you want to become another stress statistic, and join the ranks of workers in the United States who already put in more than hours on the job every year—that's 350 hours more than the Germans and slightly more than the Japanese.

How Can You Tell You Are Stressed?

Do you feel like a hamster running around on your wheel? Do you have trouble calming down, and is your body in a constant state of alert?

Seven Common Signs of Stress and Their Dangers

1. You suffer unexplained aches and pains, maybe an old injury resurfaces, or you develop a backache. Nervous tension affects all muscles and joints. During your day, as pressure builds up, your body stiffens, and you experience headaches, back pain, neck pain, or indigestion.

2. You find it difficult to concentrate at work. Your in-box is full and you dread going through your pile of work or checking your in-box because you are worried you may have missed something important.

3 You lack energy. You fret. You feel constantly tired and fatigued. Continuous worry drains you, and you are too worn out to do something physical, even though you know it will boost your energy.

4 You feel drained, frustrated, and even resentful by the demands placed on you. You may be caring for an elderly parent and raising a young child at the same time. You feel as if you don't have enough hands to do everything and find it difficult to express your feelings or ask for support.

5 Your heart beats faster and harder, which causes your pulse rate and blood pressure to rise. This can lead to heart failure and high blood pressure.

6 You can't slow down and have trouble switching off your brain. Your whole body is constantly on overdrive, and your mind is always racing. This leads to mental fatigue, eye strain, and in more serious cases, migraines and even memory loss.

7 No matter what you want to do, you don't have the energy to turn things around. You feel as if you are stuck in a rut.

> **STRESS-FREE YOGA TIP**
>
> Learning to recognize stress and anxiety
> in your life helps you feel more in control
> and on top of things.

Stress Kills. What Can You Do to Turn Your Life Around?

What can you do to relax and de-stress, have more time for yourself and your family, or simply be more creative and alert at work?

When friends or loved ones ask you "how are you feeling?" do you grumble about how tough life is, and gaze wistfully into the future, dreaming of your next vacation?

Wouldn't it be lovely if you could capture that "Happy-Feel-Good-Vacation Feeling" anytime you wanted to? Just imagine. Monday morning or doing-late night shopping on a Friday evening and in two minutes, you are at your favorite holiday destination. Just like that. No bags to pack, no airport and check-in hassles, no last-minute panicking and searching for your passport or looking for someone to water your plants. Wouldn't you like that? To feel happy, cheerful and relaxed.

Well, believe it or not, you can. It is possible to recapture the calm and tranquility you seek. Even when you are knee-deep in debt, have the gas bill to pay, and are hearing rumors of layoffs. It's still possible to be worry-free and calm.

What Can Yoga Do for You?

If you are new to yoga, do you wonder what yoga is and wonder how it can help you worry less and regain the balance between your work and personal life?

I have three creative, teenage daughters, run my own business, and have a hectic home life. Like you, I have had my fair share of life challenges—divorce, miscarriage, financial worries, bereavement, and loss. Yet, through all of this, yoga has helped me overcome my sorrow, face my pain, smile and heal.

Top Three Ways Yoga Can Help to Relieve Stress

For most of my yoga students, stress occurs when they are caring for their family and managing demanding work schedules.

Through regular yoga practice, the following three changes are the main benefits many students experience.

1. Relief from lower back pain, ease of muscle aches, improved flexibility and more energy during the day.

2. Easier to focus and be calm at work.

3. Ability to relax and worry less about things which they can't control.

Now that you see some of the benefits my yoga students experience, the following chapter shows you a few basic yoga exercises you can do at home or at work, to reduce aches and pains, relax, and energize your body.

2

STRESS TO SUCCESS

Simple Yoga Stretches to Relax and Energize Your Body

HAVE YOU EVER felt exhausted and afraid to go to work?

> **CASE STUDY:**
>
> I recall a yoga student, Catherine, a forty-year-old, female systems analyst in corporate IT. Her department was going through a major internal investigation. Catherine's job was on the line. Her best friend noticed that Catherine was drinking more coffee and taking more work home to keep on top of affairs. She recommended Catherine start yoga. The investigation lasted over nine months.
>
> *cont/d...*

> At the end of the investigation, Catherine told me her daily yoga stretches and deep breathing exercises enabled her to keep her head together, stay focused and lead her team successfully through the enquiry.

Perhaps you are going through a similar complicated time at work and are desperate for a way to relieve yourself of the constant worry and pressure.

In this chapter, you will learn and practice some of the exercises my yoga student Catherine used to help her manage her stress levels at work, during this period.

You will discover how easy it is to wake up refreshed and energized, how to be enthusiastic about life even on days when you feel overwhelmed and stressed; you will find easy, seated exercises you can do at your workstation, which are ideal to help improve your posture, relieve the ache in your lower back, loosen tight shoulders, and ease neck pain.

And at the end of the day, there are six super-fun, relaxing yoga poses you can do with your family to soothe your frazzled nerves, which means you can unwind and have a peaceful evening at home before slipping into bed.

So, if you are feeling confused, frustrated, and pressed for time, believe it or not, this is the ideal time to stop what you are doing. Take a deep breath, and do these stress-relieving yoga postures. They will leave you feeling refocused, refreshed, and better able to deal with the tension and hassles you are going through.

Gentle Reminder

If you haven't exercised for a while or have a medical condition, please consult your doctor before starting any of the practices mentioned in this book.

cont/d...

> And when you practice these yoga exercises, breathing techniques and meditation practices, please be respectful, listen to your body and be kind to yourself.
> You may think you don't have the space to do yoga at work or the time to stretch in the morning. Yet, yoga is so versatile and adaptable, you will be amazed at how easily you can fit the following yoga stretches into your busy schedule.

Top Three Ways Yoga Releases Anxiety and Boosts Your Energy

1. Yoga exercises stretch your body. As you stretch, you help to re-align and rebalance your energy body. This releases blocked energy and creates space in your body for your body to breathe.

2. Yoga poses stimulate and strengthen your "agni." Agni is your inner fire, and it is concentrated around your solar plexus. A strong inner fire helps you to digest your food well and brings vital energy into your body.

3. Yoga exercises improve your posture. When you are tired and lack energy, your body tends to sag, and you round your shoulders. As you stretch, you release and lengthen tight back and neck muscles. You feel lighter and look taller.

Now let's look at some easy yoga stretches you can do at home or at work to ease aches and pains, to relax your mind, and to nourish and energize your body.

> **Yoga for Beginner's Tip:**
> In yoga, you usually take 3-7 slow and deep breaths in and out through your nose before you start your practice. And once your mind settles, you take a steady breath in through your nose start the exercise.
> This process is known as "leading with your breath" and instantly release stress, and prepares your mind and body for the lesson.

Ntathu's Gentle, Five Yoga-in-Bed Stretches to Ease You into Your Day

As you wake, stay on your back in bed to practice these 5 yoga stretches. You will feel refreshed, balanced and focused, ready to start your day in a positive frame of mind.

1 Lying on your back, take a gentle steady breath in through your nose, and slowly breathe out through your mouth.

Repeat this 3-5 times.

Slowly raise both arms above your head, and stretch out through your fingers. Straighten your legs out on the bed.

Point and flex your toes back and forth five to seven times.

2 Squeeze your right knee to your chest. Let your left leg lay straight on the bed. Place both hands on your right shin, and gently hug your knee to your chest. Focus your awareness on your right feet, and slowly rotate your right ankle five times in one direction, relax, and repeat five times in the opposite direction.

Release your hands from your shin, straighten your right leg, and repeat this exercise with your left leg.

3 Hug both knees to your chest. Curl your body up into a small ball. Rock gently from side to side five to seven times, back and forth to each side.

Lower your head to the bed, still holding your knees to your chest, take three to five deep breaths in and out through your nose. Gently move your knees from side to side, giving a careful wringing action to the back muscles. Lower your feet back to the bed, and slowly straighten your legs on the bed.

4 Take a deep breath in, and as you exhale, slowly turn your head to look to your left shoulder. Inhale, and turn your head to the center, exhale, and turn your head to look over your right shoulder. Repeat three to five times to each side.

5 Place your left hand over your navel area and your right hand on your upper chest. Close your eyes, and take a slow steady breath in through your nose, focusing on sensing the movement of the breath, in your belly, and sending that breath all the way up to your right hand.

Repeat this belly-breathing cycle for 3-5 rounds and then slowly return to normal breathing. Be still for a few more moments, enjoying the sense of peace and inner calm. Slowly get out of bed, and begin your day.

Yoga for Beginner's Tip:

Any time you feel stressed and overwhelmed during the day, turn your attention to your breath.
Take three to five rounds of slow, steady, breaths in through your nose and out through your mouth.
This allows much more oxygen to reach your brain and body, which is the key to energizing your body and increasing vitality.

Ntathu's Eight Easy Yoga Exercises to Ease Neck and Shoulder Pain, and Release Stiffness in Your Lower Back while at Work

If your work involves sitting down all day, working at a computer, looking at a screen, chances are your shoulders ache. At the end of the day, you will notice how stiff and sore your body feels.

Yoga is great exercise for back sufferers.

The following eight easy, seated exercises can be done at your desk without any equipment or changing your clothes.

They will give your body an overall stretch and help to release neck pain, stiffness, and tension in your lower back.

> **Yoga for Beginner's Tip:**
> Before you begin these simple yoga exercises, sit comfortably on your chair.
> Place your feet flat on the floor, with your toes pointing forward.
> Rest your hands gently in your lap.
> Smile, and lower your shoulders.
> Lengthen your spine.
> Breathe slowly and deeply in and out through your nose.

Stretch and practice the following eight easy, seated, yoga exercises three to four times during your day to relieve tension, and refresh and revitalize your body and mind.

1 FEET AND ANKLES STRETCH

Sit comfortably on your chair. Make sure you sit up with a straight back.

Stretch your legs out, and slowly rotate your ankles and feet five times in each direction.

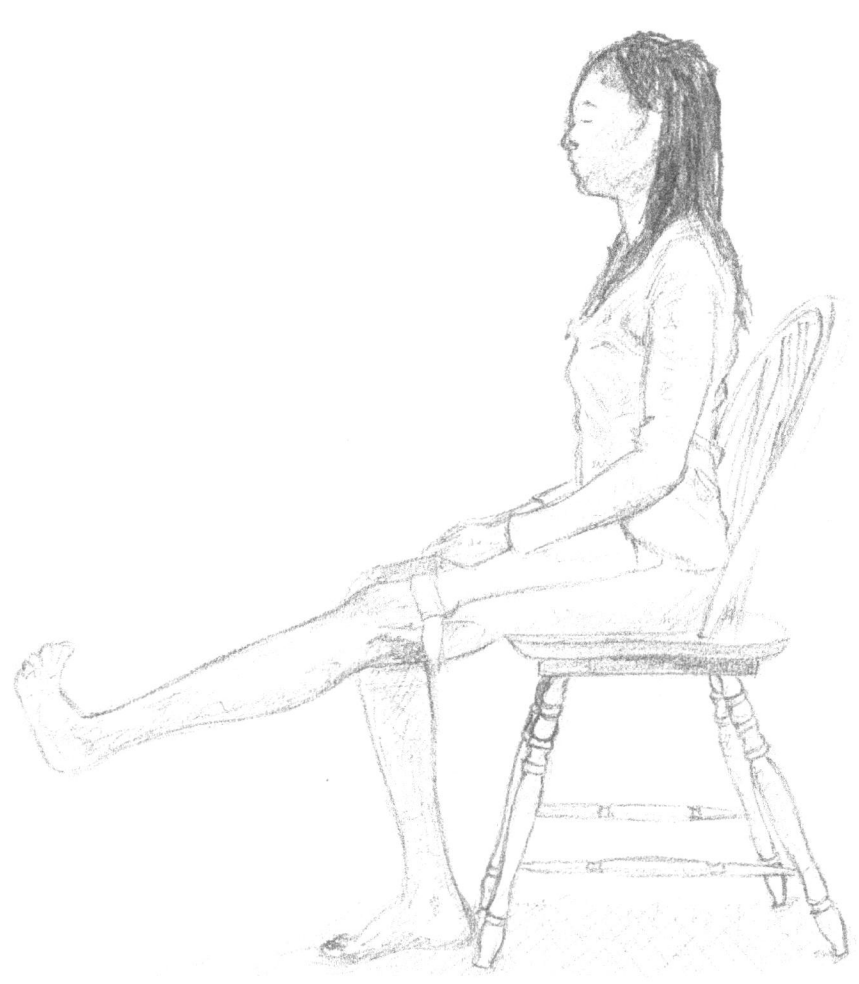

2 NECK STRETCH

Sit tall and straight; rest your hands on your lap.

Breathe in, and as you breathe out, slowly lower your right ear to your right shoulder.

Ease into the stretch, and gently return your head to center.

Repeat on the other side.

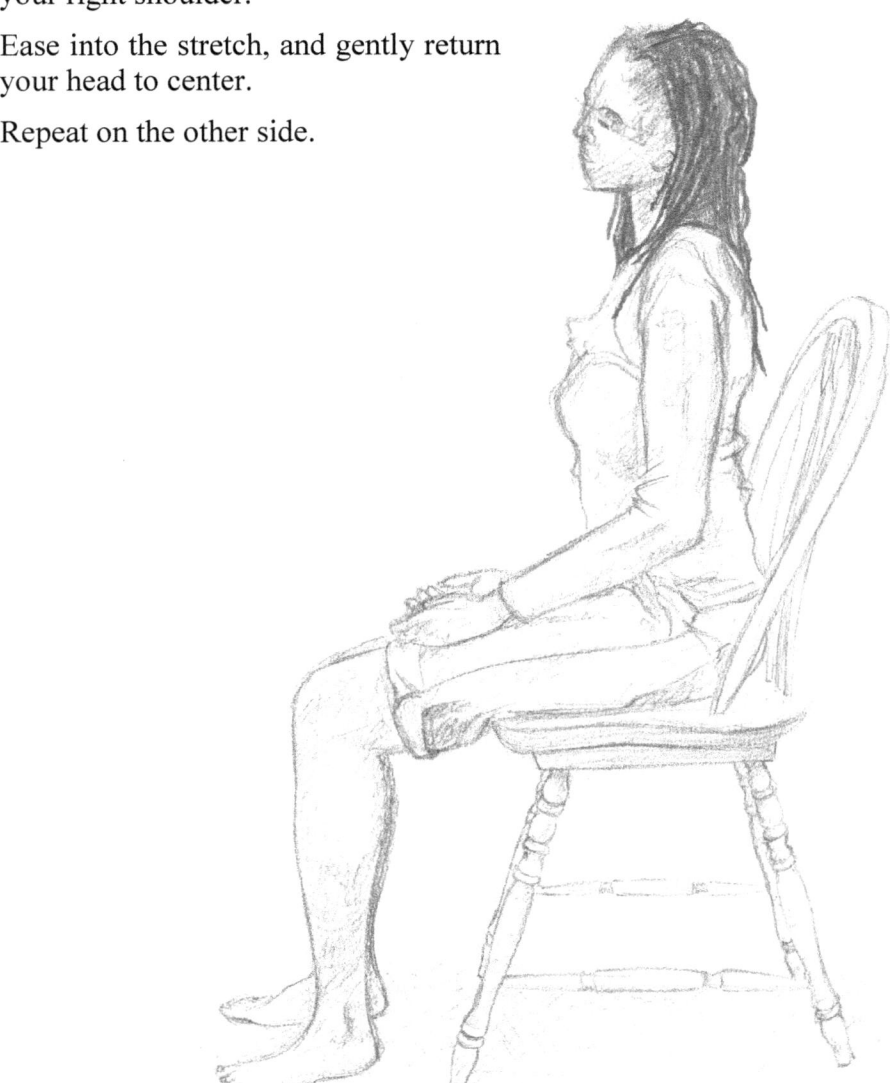

3 STRETCH ARMS ABOVE YOUR HEAD

Sitting or standing, raise both arms above your head, and stretch out through your fingers.

Hold your left wrist with your right hand, and gently stretch over to your right.

Relax and breathe into the stretch. Return to the center.

Switch arms, and repeat the exercise on the other side.

4 STRAIGHT ARM STRETCH ABOVE HEAD

Breathe in, and slowly stretch your arms up in the air above your head.

Slowly breathe out, and arch your back slightly.

Breathe in, and as you breathe out, slowly return your arms to your thighs. Repeat three to five times.

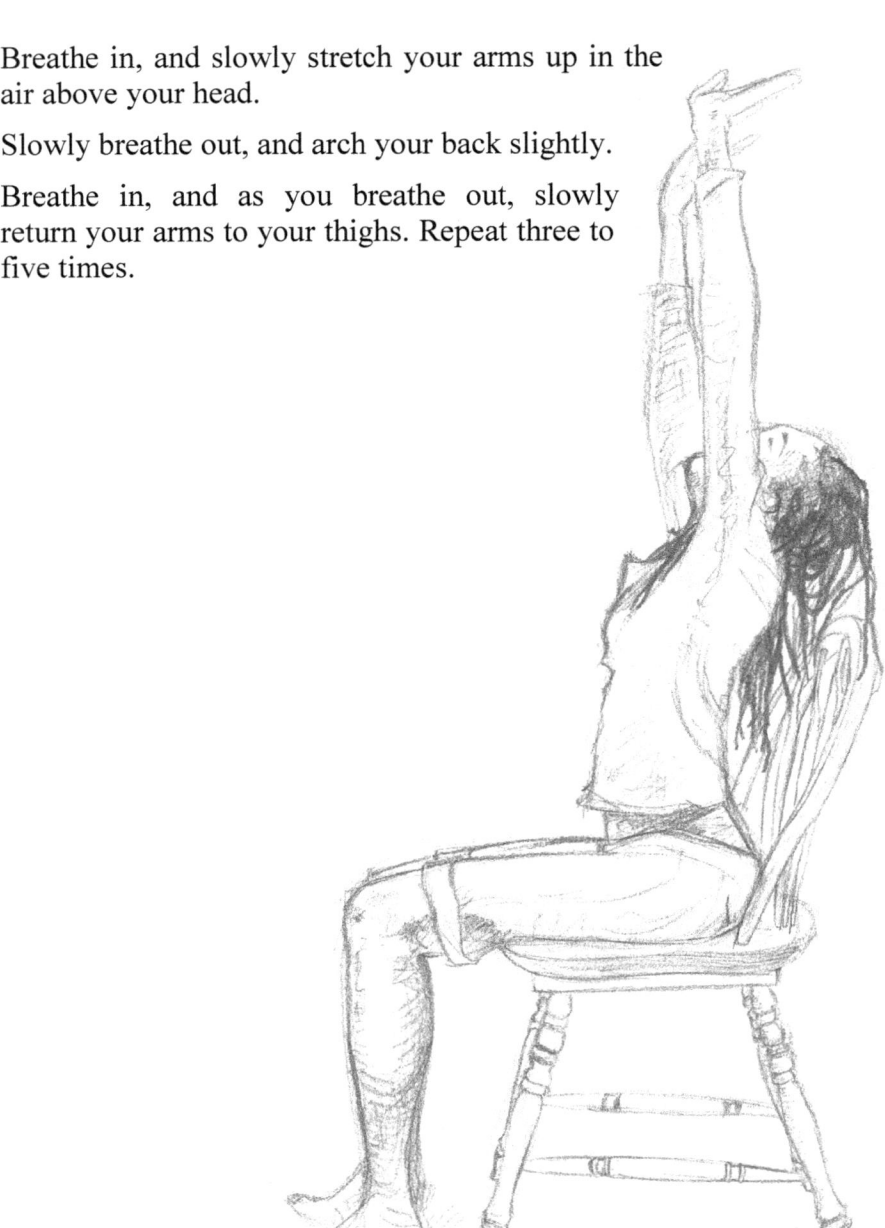

5 SEATED FORWARD BEND

Sitting on your chair, feet firmly placed on the floor, breathe in, and as you breathe out, slowly bend your upper body forward toward the ground like a rag doll.

Relax, and take three to five deep breaths before slowly returning to an upright position.

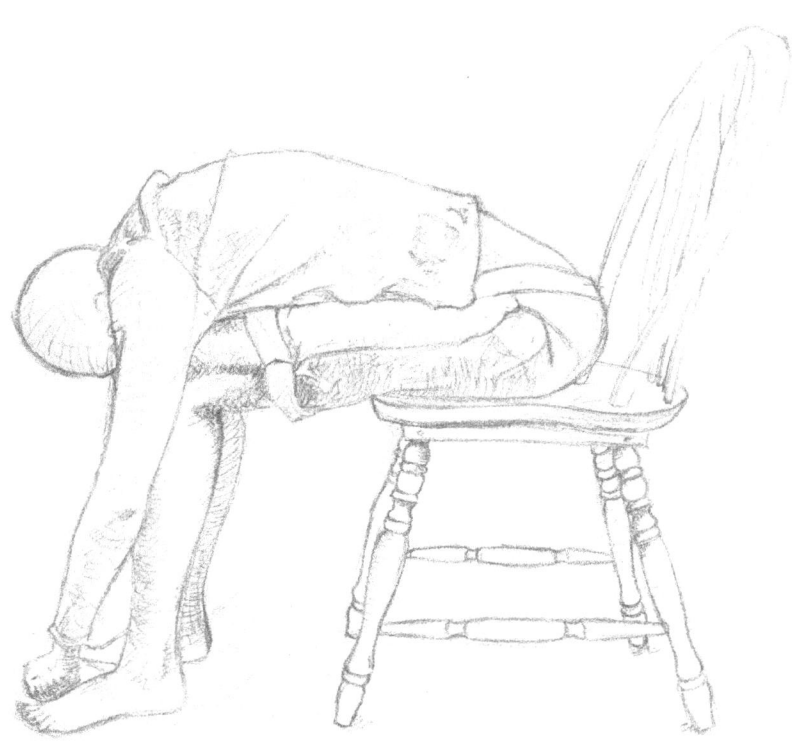

6 BACKWARD BEND

Sit comfortably on the edge of your chair.

Make sure your feet are facing forward and resting squarely on the floor.

Rest your palms on your thighs.

Breathe in, and as you breathe out, gently lift your chest, tilt your chin up as you lower your head back, and arch backward. Breathe deeply, and relax.

Slowly return your body to center.

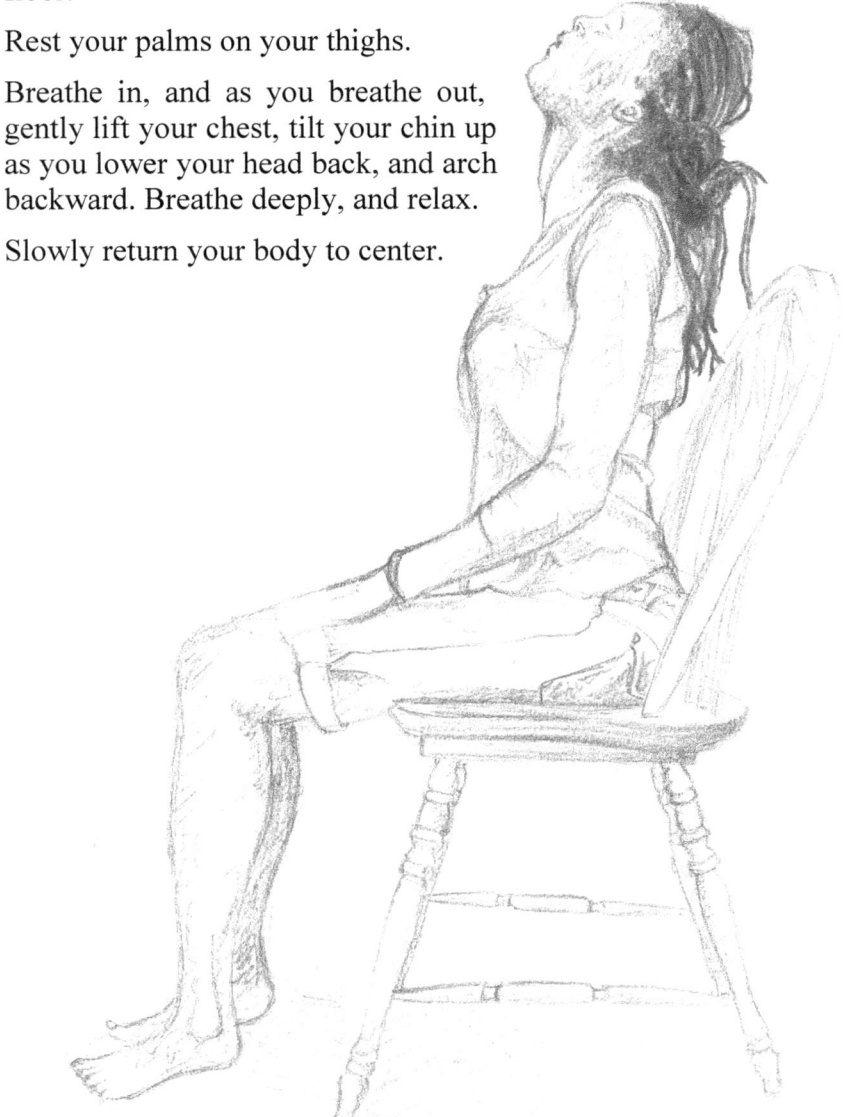

7 SEATED TRUNK TWIST

Rest your hands on your shoulders and gently twist your body side to side.

Twist slowly, three to five times in each direction.

Make sure you twist from the base of your spine, and keep your back straight throughout the stretch.

8 SEATED SPINAL TWIST

Sitting on your chair, cross your left leg over your right leg.

Place your right hand on your crossed knee.

Keeping your back straight, slowly turn your body to the left, and look over your shoulder.

Gently release, and turn back to the center.

Change legs, and twist the other way.

Rest your hands on your thighs, close your eyes, and take three to five rounds of soft, gentle breaths.

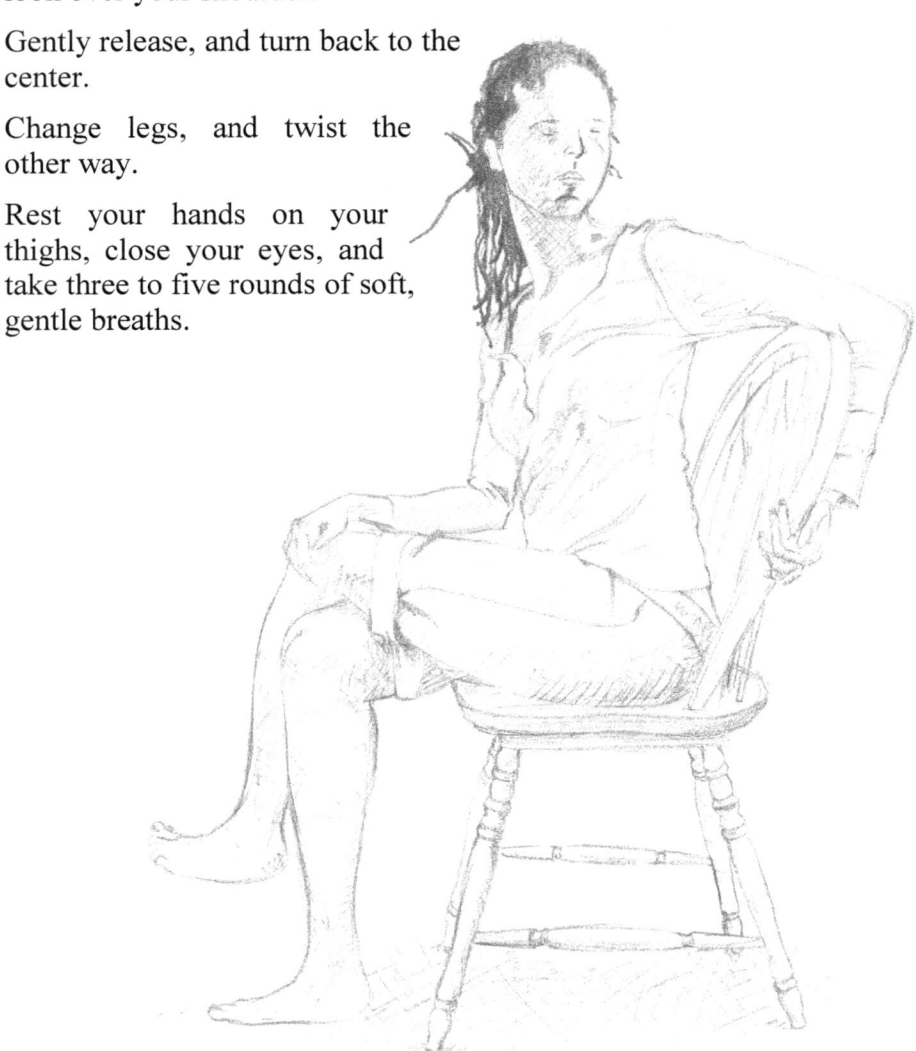

Ntathu's Six Super-Fun and Relaxing Family Yoga Poses to Help You Unwind and Calm Your Mind When Home from Work

At the end of a long day, it can be easy to grab a take-away on the way home, and collapse in front of the TV. You may dream of coming home, spending fun time with your children, or doing something with your partner, but when you get in, you are drained, worn-out and, and just want a cup of tea and nap on the settee.

Much as you want to chat with your children and spend quality family time, you feel too tired and don't have the patience or energy to listen to them and to do anything together. It is far easier for you, to order a take-away meal or heat something up in the microwave, sit on the couch, and watch TV as you eat dinner.

If you value family time and want to have fun with your family, then it is essential you learn how to relax, unwind and release tension, so you feel refreshed and have energy to enjoy being with loved ones.

Practice this super fun yoga sequence, by yourself or with your family.

This will put you in a peaceful mode for dinner; plus, you'll have fun together and feel ready to enjoy the rest of your evening.

> **Yoga for Beginner's Tip:**
> Be gentle, and never force any movements or overstretch your body. If you have a back injury, seek medical advice before doing these exercises. Always rest, and stop stretching if you feel any pain or discomfort.

1. HUGGING KNEES TO CHEST/SPINAL MASSAGE

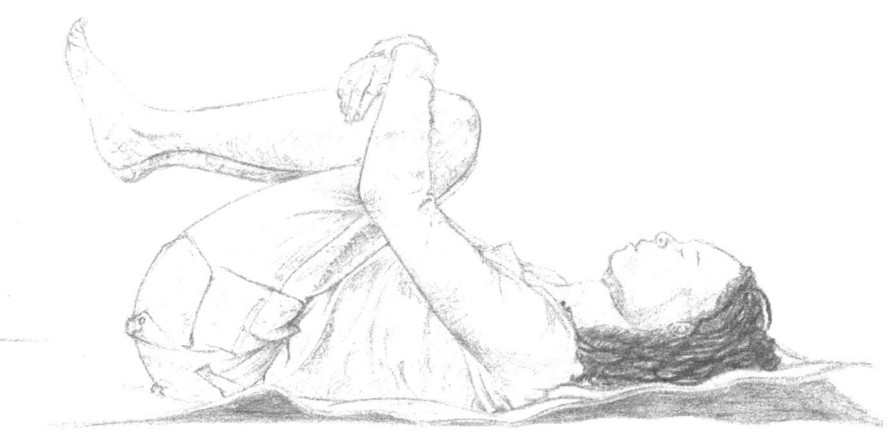

| BENEFITS: | Reduces stiffness in your lower back
Lengthens the spine
Improves flexibility |
|---|---|

Lie on your back on a comfortable surface—a yoga mat, for example.

Turn your attention to your breath, and softly breathe in through your nose and slowly breathe out through your mouth.

Hug your knees to your chest.

Keep your chin slightly tucked, so your neck is lengthened on the floor.

Hold the position as you focus on your breath, taking long and steady breaths in and out through your nose.

Next, stay in same position and rotate your knees, as if you are drawing circles with them.

Do these five to ten times in each direction.

Breathe out as the knees come close to your body, and breathe in as you move them away from your body.

Stretch your legs along the floor and rest a while.

If you are feeling more adventurous, lie on your back, hug your knees to your chest.

Roll your body from side to side, allow your elbows and the sides of your legs to touch the floor.

Roll to the right and then to the left. Be gentle, and repeat five to ten times.

Slowly unwind, and rest on your back.

Case Study:
Yoga for Back Pain Relief

My father is 83 years old. For as long as I can remember, Dad has had back pain. But, being Dad, he would ignore it and carry on with his work, or maybe take a few painkillers. He spent his life working as a mechanic, and in his spare time, his hobbies included gardening and playing cricket—all of which took their toll on his body.

As my interest in yoga grew, I introduced Dad to this pose. He regularly practices this exercise, as he says it gives him relief and eases the stiffness and pain in his back.

If you have back pain, maybe this exercise could do the same for you.

Yoga for Beginner's Tip:

Keep your shoulders lowered throughout the "hugging knees-to-chest" pose. It is easy to hunch your shoulders up to your ears, and tense your jaw as you curl up.

2 SEATED FORWARD BEND

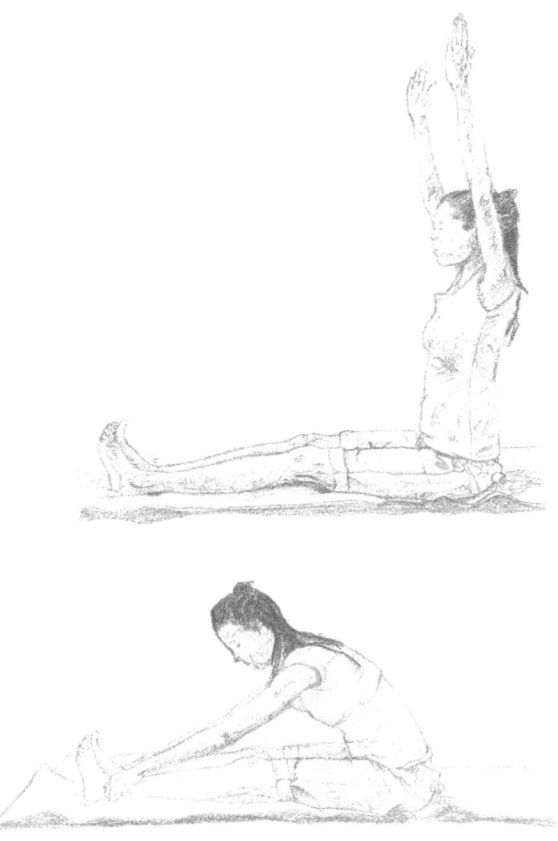

BENEFITS:	Helps to calm and quiet your mind
	Stretches your spine, hamstrings, and calves—great stretch for people who stand on their feet all day or do a lot of walking

Sit on the floor with your back straight and your legs stretched out in front of you.

Breathe in. Raise your arms straight above your head.

Breathe out. Gently bend forward at your hips, lowering your chest toward your knees.

Place your hands on your ankles or shins, whichever feels comfortable for you.

Do three to five rounds of deep breathing.

Keep your shoulders lowered, and make certain your jaw is relaxed.

Breathe in. Raise your arms straight up above your head as you sit up.

Breathe out, and lower your arms to your sides.

> **Yoga Parenting Tip:**
> If you are doing this routine with your child, as your child eases forward, gently stroke her back with a soft loving touch. This lets her know you are there, gives a beautiful massage, and helps her to relax deeper into the stretch.
> The "seated forward bend" is my favorite yoga pose. I find it great to settle my nerves, especially when my head feels "foggy," and I have been rushing around all day.

> **Yoga for Beginner's Tip:**
> Bring the chest—not your head—toward your legs. If it feels comfortable, keep your legs straight and the backs of your knees on the ground without locking your knees. Keep your feet together and toes touching the ground.

3 COBRA POSE

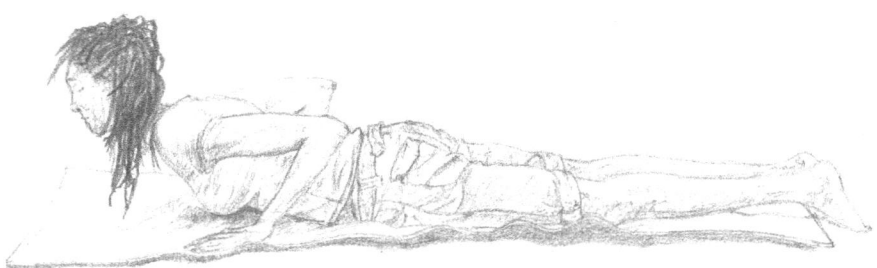

BENEFITS: Promotes flexibility and suppleness of the lower back.

Expands and opens your rib cage, allows you to breathe deeply into your abdomen.

All the abdominal organs are massaged, your appetite is stimulated, and constipation is relieved.

Yoga Parenting Tip:

Children love this pose. It resembles a cobra with its hood raised.

If you are doing this pose with your children, encourage them to hiss like a snake.

PLEASE NOTE:

Do not practice this pose if you are pregnant.

Lie on your front on your yoga mat.

Bend your elbows, and place your hands flat on the floor beneath your shoulders. Stretch your legs out flat behind you.

Tilt your head forward until your forehand touches the floor.

Tuck your elbows into your sides.

Inhale, and slowly raise your forehead, nose, and chin.

Push down with your arms, and raise your chest up, gently arching backward away from the floor.

Keep your hips and legs in contact with the floor, elbows bent and tucked into your sides.

Keep your shoulders lowered and your belly on the floor, so you get the maximum stretch of your spine.

Perform three to five rounds of deep breathing during this pose.

Exhale, and slowly lower your body to the floor.

Case Study:
Practice the Cobra for Emotional Relief

One of my beginner yoga students, Mary, at age 33, found the cobra pose ideal to release emotional hurt following her divorce. She loved the sense of ease it gave her when she breathed slowly and deeply into her heart center. Mary said whenever she came home from work, she would kick off her shoes, drop her bag, and stretch into this pose. The Cobra pose made her feel open and gave her a deep sense of relief as she breathed and let go of the tiredness of the day and sadness she felt.

If you are going through an emotionally demanding time, this pose may well be the one to help you regain your strength and inner confidence.

> **Yoga for Beginner's Tip:**
>
> If you suffer from back pain or stiffness in your lower back, keep your forearms on the floor, and keep your elbows bent throughout the pose. When you feel stronger, practice the full pose.
>
> Follow the Cobra pose with the Child's pose to rest your back.

4   CHILD'S POSE

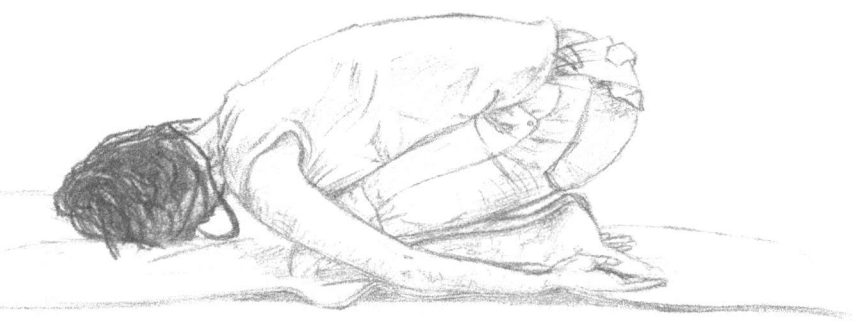

BENEFITS: A soothing pose to gently release and stretch your back and calm your nerves.

Yoga Parenting Tip:

Practice this pose with your child. It gives a feeling of safety and privacy. Encourage them to pretend they are a rock and be very still and quiet, or they can be a mouse, and squeak as they rest in the pose.

When my daughters were younger and feeling restless, I would encourage them to curl up in "the mouse pose," as I gently rocked and stroked their back. After a while, they'd drift off and wake up a few minutes later, relaxed and re-energized.

Kneel with your big toes touching, heels slightly apart.

Make sure you feel comfortable on your heels.

Lean forward, and rest your forehead on the ground.

Place your arms by your sides next to your body, palms facing upward, fingers pointing back toward your feet.

Stay still and take three to five slow, deep breaths.

Soften and relax your whole body as you breathe gently in and out through your nose for as long as you feel comfortable.

One Older Student Named Judy says:

*"My knees are a bit stiff and inflexible,
so I rest my forehead on top of my fists."*

Yoga for Beginner's Tip:

Keep your weight resting on your heels, not on your head. Your head is a resting point, not a support.
If you find the child pose causes pain in your knees and hips, roll over onto your back.
Gently hug your knees to your chest (see hugging knees to chest pose).
This has the similar stretching effect on your spine.

5 COBBLER POSE

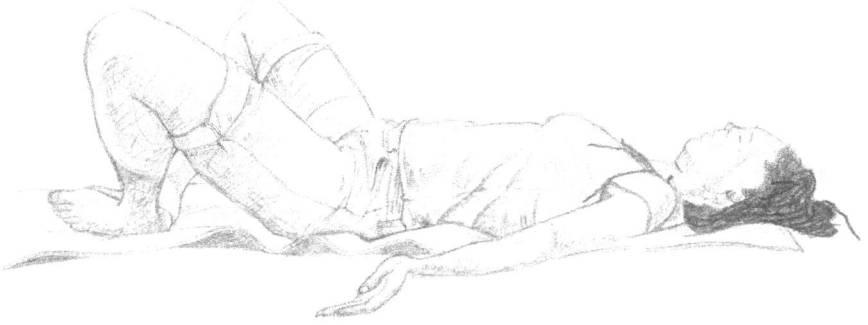

BENEFITS: Helps to open the hip joints and release tension from your pelvis.
Stretches inner thighs and hips.
Excellent pose to practice during menstruation and pregnancy, especially if you focus on breathing deeply into your belly and send positive affirmations to your womb.

Case Study:
Loosen Stiff Hips

One of my yoga students, Anna, is 69 years old and has very stiff hips. Anna came to yoga to improve her posture, improve her sense of balance, and gain suppleness in her hips.
Regular practice of the Tree Pose and Cobbler Pose helped Anna achieve these goals.
She now walks with a loose gait, feels taller, and can move without feeling so stiff in her hip region.

Lie down on your back—if you wish, you can place a bolster cushion along the length of your spine—and bring the soles of your feet together close to your body with your knees open wide.

Allow your knees to sink toward the floor, and focus on breathing gently yet deeply into your belly.

Enjoy the gentle stretch along your inner thighs.

In this position, you can also bring your arms over your head and loosely clasp your hands. Or you can rest your hands-on top of your belly and focus on the rising and falling of your abdomen as you breathe in and out.

Keep your lower back pressed down toward the floor.

Breathe deeply three to five times.

To come out of the pose, bring your arms back down to the sides of your body, and slowly straighten your legs.

Yoga for Beginner's Tip:

If your back and hips are very inflexible, lean against a wall, and place a cushion in between the floor and your lower back. This makes it easier for you to focus on softening and opening your hips.

Stress-free Parenting Tip:

While in the Cobbler pose, you can encourage your child to be a butterfly. Invite your child to gently flap their knees and wave their arms like butterflies.
Ask your child, "What color are your wings today…?"
I love to practice the Butterfly/Cobbler pose with children; they have such vivid imaginations!
I am always amazed at how bold, colorful, sparkly, and bright their wings are.
I remember one small boy had Superman wings, and another girl had the most adorable rainbow-colored wings dotted with drops of sunshine-yellow and splashes of pink bubbles…
Wow… I wonder what color your wings are…

6 LEAN ON ME/BACK-TO-BACK BREATHING EXERCISE

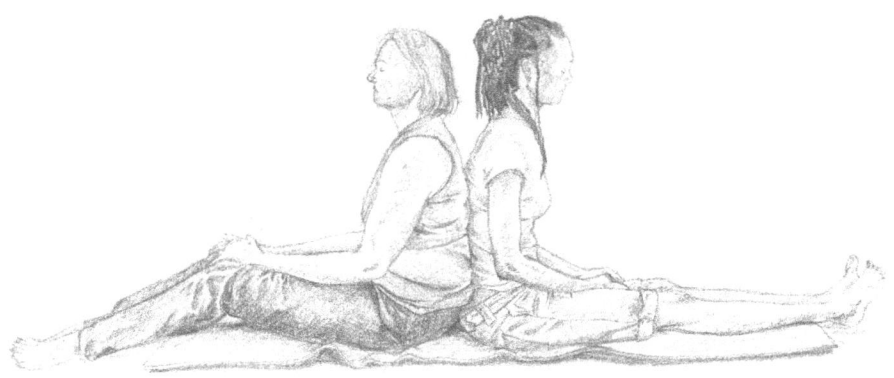

At the end of your "family yoga time," Lean on Me helps to bring a sense of harmony and stillness to the end of the session.

Sit on the floor back-to-back with either your child or your partner.

You can sit cross-legged, or stretch your legs out along the floor.

Close your eyes.

Become aware of your breathing, and gently sway from side to side with your partner, as both of you grow calm.

Then be still, and just lean against your partner, feeling the warmth and stability from supporting each other.

Stay as long as you both feel comfortable.

Slowly open your eyes, turn around, and give each other a hug and smile.

Yoga for Beginner's Tip:

Make sure both of you keep your back upright and touching as much as possible…all the way along the length of your spine.

Yoga Parenting Tip:

Use this exercise to totally calm down and reconnect with your child/partner. As you gently sway from side to side, remind yourself of the joys, fun, and blessings you and your child/partner give to each other.

BEDTIME RITUAL

Do you have trouble falling asleep at night?

Do you have trouble sleeping? Have you ever awakened, feeling troubled and exhausted from lack of sleep? Maybe your sleep is disturbed because your partner snores.

Lack of sleep tends to leave you feeling crabby with loved ones, and it may even affect your capability to concentrate while driving or at work. If you have had a demanding day at work, it can be difficult for you to "switch off" when you come home. Staying up late at night, watching television, or eating late overstimulates your brain. No wonder you can't unwind and fall asleep!

How Can I Get a Good Night's Sleep Without Drugs?

To get a good night's sleep, especially if you have had stressful day, it is essential for you to find a way to unwind and calm your mind before you go to bed.

Simple breathing and gentle yoga exercises are great ways to help soothe your mind, and prepare your body for a restful night of sleep. After you practice these stretches, notice how you sleep so much better and awaken refreshed and rejuvenated.

Here's Five Ways to Get a Good Night's Sleep Without Drugs

1 Sit comfortably with a straight spine and your feet firmly resting on the floor. Close your eyes, and take a long, steady breath in through your nose, and then slowly breathe out through your nose. Do this three more times, as it helps to calm and clear your mind. Next, breathe in slowly for a count of three, and then slowly breathe out for a count of six. Repeat this sequence of breathing in for three seconds and out for six seconds, three to seven times. Slowly open your eyes, and be aware of how calm and relaxed you feel.

2. Give yourself a hand and finger massage. Gently massage your fingers and thumbs. Take time to really enjoy your mini hand massage. If you have a favorite hand cream or even warm olive oil, use it to add a bit of luxury to your evening.

3. Brush/stroke down your left arm with your right hand. Repeat the action on the opposite arm.

Yoga for Beginner's Tip:
Remember, in yoga, relaxation is an art—a moment in time you gift to yourself.

4. Practice the Seated Rag Doll pose. Simply bend at your waist and slowly fold your torso forward and downwards your thighs, keeping your feet firmly on the ground. Allow your knees to remain soft, and make sure your neck isn't stiff (the goal here is to remain soft and wobbly). Relax your jaw, and allow your arms to swing and flop from side to side. Stay in this position for one to two minutes.

5. Lie on your stomach. Fold your arms, and rest your cheek on your arms. Observe the rising and falling of your abdomen as it expands and contracts with each breath. Stay in this position, and take three to five rounds of deep, abdominal breathing.

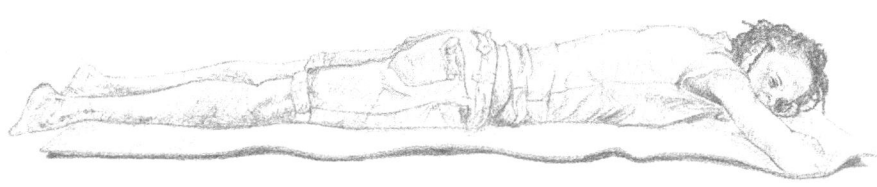

Now that you have learned how easy it is to release stress and feel relaxed and energized, turn to the next chapter to see how quickly yoga breathing exercises can calm and quiet your mind, so you can concentrate on your daily tasks.

3

CRAZY-BUSY TO BLISSFULLY CALM

Deep-Breathing Exercises to Revitalize and Reenergize

HAVE YOU EVER been in a situation where your mind is so full of "things to do" that you feel overwhelmed and perhaps even frightened?

Maybe you have to give a presentation at work and feel anxious about speaking in front of your colleagues.

Worry, a form of fear and anxiety, creates tension in your body.

When you are stressed, you aren't operating at your full capacity. If you continue to worry, your work suffers, your health may deteriorate, and you might find it difficult to make good decisions and get things done.

In this chapter, you will discover why yoga breathing is so important. You'll learn how to revitalize, replenish, and reenergize your system through your breath. You'll discover whether you breathe correctly and learn various breathing exercises.

Once you begin using these as part of your daily routine, half your worries will disappear, or, at the very least, things won't worry you quite as much.

What Happens When You Breathe Correctly?

On a basic level, breathing allows you to draw oxygen into your body and eliminate toxins and bacteria that impede your body's ability to function correctly.

As a yoga teacher, I regularly see students who report the benefits of using the yoga breathing exercises. They apply the exercises they've learned in class when they feel anxious or unsure of themselves. For example, they might practice these breathing exercises just before working directly with their team manager, before meeting new people at a network conference, or even before attending the annual family gathering.

The slower and deeper you can breathe, the more oxygen you'll allow to enter and flow through your body. This expands your lung capacity and stimulates and opens your heart, which instantly makes you feel more confident, brighter, and happier.

> **Yoga for Beginner's Tip**
> Do you know the power of your breath?
> Learning how to breathe correctly is one of the most important lessons you will learn when you incorporate yoga techniques to create a stress-free life.

From a yogic perspective, your breath is the link between your mind and your body. When you learn to control your breathing, you align your mind with your body; your body becomes steady, and you experience inner peace and calm.

Learning to breathe well is a skill.

You may be surprised to realize that your breath is directly linked to your body. Understanding the link between the mind and body connection enables you to look at ways you can improve your health. When you breathe deeply and fully, you activate the parasympathetic nervous system. This allows the rest and digest response to filter through your body—as opposed to the fight or flight stress response that generally governs your life.

> **Yoga for Beginner's Tip:**
> Traditionally, yoga breathing exercises form the core of yoga. Known as *pranayama*, deep-breathing exercises, form the link between your mind and body.
> Deep breathing exercises, especially when combined with mindful movement, helps to stimulate the parasympathetic nervous system, which promotes calm.

What Happens to Your Breath When You Are Angry?

Have you noticed that when you are tense, your breath is fast and shallow, or you may even hold your breath when you're anxious?

When you are angry, your breathing is rapid and sharp, or when you are depressed and sad, your breathing is uneven and slightly jumpy. Conversely, when you are relaxed, happy, and joyful, your breathing is slow and even. This is the ideal way to breathe.

> **Yoga for Beginner's Tip:**
> There is a saying in yoga that we come into this world with an allocated number of breaths, and it is not the number of years lived that determine the length of your life but the number of breaths taken. Therefore, it is vital you learn how to breathe correctly to maximize your lifespan.

Why Yoga Breathing is So Important

Learning how to breathe correctly can help you manage the negative effects of distress—for example, headaches, stomach disorders, fatigue, insomnia, and weight gain.

Everyone suffers from nervous tension and anxiety at some time in their life. You might be going through a painful divorce or mourning the loss of a close relative or friend. You might even be facing disciplinary action at work or recovering from major surgery. All these incidents affect your immune system, which in turn can lower your ability to stay vital and on top of things.

> **Yoga Parenting Tip:**
> Breathing exercises can help your child to listen and concentrate better at school—especially if they are fidgety and restless. Teens can practice deep breathing prior to taking exams to help calm their nerves and improve their focus.

Seven Simple Steps to Deep Breathing Correctly to Calm Your Nerves

1. Lie on your back on your bed or on a yoga mat. Make sure you feel comfortable.

2. Straighten your legs out along the bed (unless you have a bad back or pain in your lower back, in which case, you should bend your knees and have your feet flat on the bed or mat).

3. Place your hands on your belly. Cradle your belly with your hands, and allow the fingertips of both hands to lightly touch each other.

4. Close your eyes, and start to turn your attention to focusing on your breath. Don't try to control your breathing; just breathe slowly and gently, noticing how you are breathing, as you softly breathe in and out through your nose.

5. Slowly breathe in for a count of four—in through your nose—and then breathe out for a count of four, again through your nose. You will notice your belly and hands rise and fall with each breath.

Repeat this pattern of breathing, in and out, five to ten times.

Slowly open your eyes, and be aware of how calm, relaxed and focused you feel.

Yoga for Beginner's Tip:

Take one-minute, "deep-breathing breaks" throughout your day, during which you close your eyes and consciously tune into how you're breathing.

This enables you to reduce the build-up of pressure, calm and clear your mind, and boost your energy - all positive steps toward feeling vital and well.

Wake Up with a Zing. A Simple, Deep-Breathing Exercise to Help You Feel Invigorated and Alive

Have you even lain in bed, exhausted, one eye on the clock, wishing time would stop, so you could lie there forever?

Next time you wake up and feel gloomy, off balance, or just plain tired from lack of sleep, try this simple, yogic breathing exercise to ease irritability and soothe any anxiety you may be feeling.

1. Lie on your back in your bed with your eyes closed. Stretch out your legs…about twelve to eighteen inches apart. Tuck your chin slightly into your chest, which helps to ease tension from the back of your neck. Make sure you feel comfortable.

2. Rest the palm of your right hand firmly yet gently on top of your navel, and put your left hand just below your collarbone.

3. Take a slow, steady breath, in through your nose, drawing from the area beneath your right hand, and breathe slowly, following a path up to your left hand. Slowly breathe out.

4. Repeat this four to seven times, breathing slowly and deeply this way, as you feel your thoughts begin to settle.

5. Slowly release your hands, and gently stretch your body. Rest a while in your bed, and feel the calm and bliss in your body.

On a personal note, learning to breathe correctly and practicing yoga breathing exercises as soon as I woke up helped to ease the pain and sorrow I experienced as I grieved the loss of my dear brother. After John's death, I found it difficult to breathe and kept getting severe chest pains. My bereavement counsellor suggested I practice this breathing exercise. If you are grieving, you might want to try this exercise to see if it makes a difference in how you feel.

> **Yoga for Beginner's Tip:**
> People who practice yoga believe that by doing yoga breathing exercises, we become more attuned to the rhythm of the universe. This helps to reduce feelings of loneliness, anger, frustration, despair, and sadness and fosters a sense of belonging and connectedness with others.

AT WORK Two-Minute Break, Watch-your-Breathing Exercise

Most of us can take two minutes for ourselves at work now and then.

This simple, yoga breathing exercise leaves your mind feeling clear and relaxed and is ideal to do if you are stressed out, and Friday feels far away.

1. Sit on a chair in a comfortable, upright position. Set your phone's timer for two minutes. Make sure your back is straight, relax your jaw, soften your eyes, relax your shoulders, and rest your hands on your lap.

2. Breathe naturally, and watch your breath. Be aware of your inhale, and be aware of your exhale. Simply focus on your breathing. If your mind wanders and you turn to other thoughts, acknowledge the thoughts, the energy of the thoughts, and then return your awareness to your breathing.

3. Keep watching and listening to your breathing. Notice your thoughts slowing down as your body lets go of tension.

4. Sit still for at least two minutes with your mind focused on your breathing.

5. Bring your awareness back to the room slowly. Gently open your eyes, and notice how much clearer, invigorated, and relaxed you feel.

> **Yoga for Beginner's Tip:**
> Repeat this simple, yoga breathing exercise whenever you get up to take a tea or coffee break.

> **Yogic Parenting Tip:**
> Teach your child to become aware of how they breathe by letting them look at a shape or image -
> for example, a round dinner plate.
> Ask them to inhale halfway around the shape, and then exhale and complete the circle.
> Invite them to practice this three to five times in each direction.

A Breathing Exercise for Good Posture. Straight Arms Behind Back

Have you noticed how slumped and slouched you become during your day, especially if you spend most of your time working on a computer?

Just as an observation, next time you are out in the shopping mall, have a look at way other people are standing and walking and holding their body.

How many people can you see who have rounded and slumped shoulders, their head hanging at an odd angle as they use their mobile phones, or who slouch when they sit down?

What impression do you get when you see someone stand tall, straight, and proud?

Do they look self-assured, inspire confidence and trust?

My older yoga students always say how stronger and taller they feel after practicing these yoga stretches.

STRAIGHT ARMS BEHIND BACK

BENEFITS: This simple exercise is excellent for chicken neck and stooped, rounded shoulders, as it opens the chest and readily promotes deep breathing.

1. Stand straight with your feet a few inches apart. Put your hands behind your back, and interlock your fingers, palms upward. Now, turn your palms down.

2. Inhale deeply, then bend forward while exhaling. At the same time, raise your arms until they are stretched out.

3. Keep your elbows as straight as you can without causing discomfort. Keep your chin tucked in as you breathe in and out, and try to raise your arms a bit higher with each breath.

4 Stay in this position for three to five breaths. On an out-breath, slowly release your arms as you return to an upright position.

Repeat the whole exercise two or three times.

> ## Case Study:
>
> A couple of my senior yoga students, Vera and Rose, both in their sixties, love the Straight Arms Behind Back exercise, as it gives them the sense of feeling upright and tall.
>
> Initially it was difficult for them to hold their hands behind their back and raise their arms, so I encourage them just to stand and clasp their hands behind their back. With regular practice, their mobility has improved, and they are now able to raise their arms up a lot higher than before.

Six Anywhere-Anytime, Yoga Breathing Exercises to Beat Stress and Restore Energy

Learning how to recognize and manage your stress levels is essential to help you stay healthy and be happy.

> **Yoga for Beginner's Tip:**
> The practice of yogic-breathing exercises offers you a way to move through your worries and anxieties, and deal with concerns in a more cheerful and positive way. The following yoga breathing exercises are among the ones my yoga students at work regularly say give them the maximum benefit in releasing pressures. They are simple to do and can be practiced anywhere and at any time of the day when you must focus and concentrate.

One. Observe the Breath

Sit comfortably, close your eyes, and become aware of how you are breathing. Don't change your breathing, just be present, and observe the movement of air in and out through your nose.

Allow your breathing to find its own natural rhythm, and continue to listen and observe your breathing for two minutes.

When you practice this tip, at first, you might find it hard to concentrate on your breathing. Don't worry. Whenever your mind wanders or you lose concentration, just return to observing your breathing.

Two. Diaphragmatic Breathing

You can practice diaphragmatic breathing while lying down on your back on a comfortable surface, sitting comfortably in a chair, or even standing up.

> **BENEFITS:** Helps to develop concentration and balances the right and left sides of the brain.

Gently place one hand on your upper chest and the other hand on your belly.

Relax your belly and chest.

Keep your mouth closed.

Breathe in through your nose, and feel your belly, rising and expanding, then feel the ribcage rising, and finally, the upper chest.

As you exhale, feel the belly sink down.

Practice five to seven repetitions of diaphragmatic breathing, then slowly open your eyes. Be still for a few moments until you feel ready to gently re-engage with your day.

Yoga for Beginner's Tip:

Remember, when you practice yoga breathing exercises, to sit upright, relax your shoulders and lightly tuck your chin in, as this helps to keep your head, neck and back in a nice straight line.

Three. Lion Roar

Although not technically a traditional pranayama exercise, the Lion Roar is one of my yoga students' favorite breathing exercises because it is fun to do and quickly helps them release frustration and the buildup of anxiety and stress.

Sit or stand comfortably.

Scrunch up your face like a dried prune.

Open your eyes, and look upward.

Open your mouth, stretch out your tongue, and *roarrrrrr* like a lion. Repeat three times and when you've finished, smile and notice how you feel. I guarantee you'll feel better.

Yoga Parenting Tip:

Children *love* this breathing exercise.

If your child is bored or grumpy and miserable, get them up, and do the Lion Roar.

The longer they roar, the more frustration they'll release, which will make them feel happier, motivated and feel calmer.

Yoga for Beginner's Tip:

Try one of the above breathing-practice techniques anytime you feel swamped, and notice the difference it makes in your life. You will feel rejuvenated, more vitality, and will find it easier to get going to complete tasks at hand.

Special Breathing Exercise for Children—The Bumble Bee Breath

> **BENEFITS:** Fun to do and helps your child understand the power of their breathing to calm, balance, and quiet their thoughts.

Make sure your child is sitting comfortably with his or her back straight.

Ask your child to close her eyes and slowly breathe in through her nose, and then ask her to pretend she is a bumble bee and to make a long humming sound as she breathes out.

She can make a high humming sound one time and a low or soft and gentle humming sound the next.

Repeat this three to seven times.

For the last breath, encourage your child not to make any sound at all and to listen to the silence.

> **Yoga Parenting Tip:**
> Practice this exercise with your child.
> Make it a fun game, and enjoy the silence together at the end of the exercise.

Two Advanced Popular Yoga Breathing Exercises for Calm and to Improve Your Yoga Practice

The following two yoga breathing exercises, Single Nostril breathing and Alternate Nostril breathing, are offered here for more experienced yogis, who may be reading this book. They are ideal if you have practiced yoga before, go to a regular yoga class and familiar with yoga breathing exercises. Otherwise, I'd suggest, you stick with the basic breathing exercises in this book and try these two when you have more experience in practicing yoga.

Regular practice of Single Nostril breathing and Alternate Nostril breathing will encourage full, deep breathing, which, over time, strengthens your ability to hold and maintain your yoga exercises and is excellent preparation for meditation.

Single Nostril Breathing for Deep Calm

BENEFITS: A calming breathing practice, Single Nostril Breathing helps to create balance in the body. Breathing through your right nostril helps to stimulate your energy, while breathing through your left nostril calms and relaxes your emotions.
To get the most out of this breathing exercise, practice Part A in the morning and Part B in the evening before bed.

Part A: Sit in a comfortable position, spine straight, body relaxed. Rest your left hand on your lap. Turn your attention to your right hand, bend the index and middle finger into the palm. The thumb, ring and little finger are up (this position is known as *Vishnu Mudra*). The thumb is used to close the right nostril, the ring and little finger the left nostril.

Close your left nostril with your ring and little fingers. Breathe in through your right nostril for a count of four, and then slowly breathe out for a count of eight. Repeat this five to ten times. Relax, and return your right hand to your lap.

Part B: In the evening, just before you go to bed, repeat the above steps, but this time, close your right nostril, using your right thumb. Breathe in through your left nostril for a count of four, and then slowly breathe out for a count of eight. Repeat this five to ten times. Relax and return your hands to your lap. Take a few moments to sit still and notice how you feel.

> **Yoga for Beginner's Tip:**
> Breathing correctly offers you a quick tool to release tension, reduce the effects of stress on your body and to calm your mind. Yogic-breathing exercises are useful strategies to employ to support your intention to live a stress-free life.
> There are various types of yoga breathing exercises you can use as part of your daily practice or self-care routine to help you relax and reduce stress.
> One of my favorite's is Alternate Nostril breathing because it helps me to feel strong, peaceful and balanced.

What Is Alternate Nostril Breathing?

Alternate Nostril Breathing (traditionally known as Anuloma Viloma) is a classic yogic breathing exercise and practiced at the beginning or end of a yoga lesson.

When Do You Practice Alternate Nostril Breathing?

Whenever you feel out of alignment and start getting ratty and tense or feel anxious then that's a sign your energy needs to be re-aligned and rebalanced.

Alternate Nostril breathing helps with this process because it alternates the flow of breath/prana through one nostril and then the other.

How Do You Practice Alternate Nostril Breathing?

As with all yoga exercises, please listen and respect your body. Any sign of discomfort, dizziness or pain in the body, please stop, rest and if needed see your Doctor. If you are pregnant or new to yoga, I'd suggest you familiarize yourself with more basic yoga breathing exercises before trying this more advanced practice.

Simple Guidelines for The Practice Of Alternate Nostril Breathing

Traditionally Alternate Nostril breathing is practiced in the ratio of 1:4:2 -for every second/count of breath you inhale, you retain your breath for four times as long and exhale for twice as long – for example, if you inhale for a count of 2, then you hold your breath for a count of 8 and exhale for account of 4. Depending on your level of experience, you can, for example inhale for account of 4, retain for 16 and breathe out for a count of 8.

There are six steps to complete one round of Alternate Nostril Breathing

Before you start, make sure you are sitting comfortably either on a chair or cross-legged on the floor.

Sit upright with a straight spine.

Rest your back of your left hand on your left knee, with your thumb and index finger touching;

With your right hand, bend your index and middle fingers into your palm, which leaves your right thumb to close your right nostril and your ring and little fingers to close your left nostril.

Before you start, spend a few moments in quiet focusing on your everyday breath as you allow your mind and body to settle into the practice.

Exhale fully, close your right nostril with your right thumb, slowly exhale through your left nostril for a count of 4.

Gently hold your breath, by "pinching" both nostrils between your thumb and ring and little finger, for a count of 16.

Release your thumb from your right nostril (keep your left nostril closed) and exhale through your right nostril for a count of 8.

Keeping your left nostril closed, breathe in through your right nostril for a count of four.

Close both nostrils and hold your breath for a count of 16 (as in #2).

Release your left fingers from your left nostril, keep your right nostril closed with your right thumb and breathe out through the left nostril for a count of eight.

This completes one round of this practice. Aim to do between three to seven rounds.

~

Now that you've learned a few yoga and breathing exercises, would you like to discover another popular yoga technique to help you think clearly, let-go off negative thoughts and be kinder to yourself?

In the next chapter, we'll explore the power of meditation and how meditating can help you to totally appreciate the power of your breath, boost your energy, improve your decision-making skills, and best of all, give you the ability to focus and be calm during your busy day.

4

PANIC TO PEACE

The Power of Meditation to Clear Your Mind and Improve Your Happiness and Wellbeing

HOW OFTEN HAVE you longed for peace and quiet? For some time alone to rest, sit quietly and be at peace?

> **Case Study:**
>
> Carol, one of my yoga students, found it hard to relax, unwind, and switch off at the end of the day. She would lie awake at night, replaying all the mistakes she felt she had made during the day. Carol struggled to get things done at work.
>
> *cont/d...*

> Her brain felt muddled with all the pressures and demands on her. Lack of support and resources from her manager, left Carol feeling vulnerable and ill-prepared to do her job properly. At home, she found it an effort to be present and help her children with their homework. She wanted to help them with their homework, listen patiently and talk to them about their day, yet, every night, Carol found herself shouting and moaning at her children. This made her feel guilty, and she went to bed, annoyed with herself and doubting her ability to do well at work and be a "good mum". Constantly worrying about what happened at work prevented Carol from relaxing and enjoying her time at home with her children. She longed to find a way to solve the problems at work easily and smoothly and, most importantly, to spend more fun, relaxed time with her family.
>
> As with most of my new clients, Carol had heard about meditation and knew it would be good for her, yet she felt it would be too hard to learn, she didn't have time to fit anything else into her day and felt meditation was something "people like her" didn't do.

In this chapter, you will find out how meditation helped Carol and some of my other students learn how to focus, slow down their thoughts, and think more clearly. I will share with you some of the meditation techniques Carol used, which also helped her to "switch off" from work mode and finally, unwind and have a relaxed evening with her children.

Once the domain of monks and spiritual seekers, meditation has gained popularity among the general population. Doctors are now recommending meditation and mindfulness meditation to help people balance and manage their complex lives.

Why Meditate?

Finding time to develop meaningful relationships and have fun with your family can seem like a luxury, especially if you are busy and already spend a large portion of your day working hard at work.

If you can identify with Carol and you also have a crazy-busy life and you long for peace, silence and quiet then I am sure you will find meditation a useful skill to learn.

What Is Meditation?

Meditation is the process whereby you can focus and still and quieten your mind, so you feel less overwhelmed and stressed and more able to stay positive and alert during the day. During meditation, you learn to gently observe your thoughts, calm and quiet your mind and, with practice experience a deep sense of calm, clarity, and expanding awareness of your infinite potential and ability to live a more harmonious life.

Can Anyone Practice Meditation?

Yes, I believe everyone has the potential to meditate.

However, not everyone has the patience or inclination to meditate. Meditation isn't easy. The mind has been likening to chattering monkey. It takes time, love and commitment to take the time to learn how to relax the body and calm and still the mind.

Top Benefits of Meditation for Busy People

- Meditation helps to strengthen the mind.
- Meditation promotes effective breathing habits.
- Meditation gives you strength to forgive others and yourself.
- Meditation enhances your intuition and your sense of curiosity and wonder in the world.

- Meditation promotes positive and healthy thoughts.
- Meditation affirms your connection to humankind and to the joyfulness found in life.

You probably spend a large portion of your time working, and if your work/home life is anything like most people's, your day is dominated by your work. Taking care of your child or children and organizing your family life is often squeezed in between work, meetings and other social commitments.

With so many tasks to do in a day, it is easy to feel overwhelmed and stuck. In this state, it can be difficult for you to think clearly and make informed decisions. To manage your time effectively, and fit in everything you need to do, you need to have a system which gives you energy to look after your family, do your jobl, and help you care for your health and well-being.

If you are looking for a way to find inner peace, calm and quiet in your life, then the ancient art of meditation may provide you with the calm you are seeking.

What Happens When You Meditate?

Meditation has been likened to observing the sea on a clear, calm day. You sit and gaze at the horizon, and you get a glimpse of your true potential.

During meditation, your brain undergoes certain physiological changes, all of which counteract the negative effects of stress. The para-sympathetic nervous system is activated, which leads to an increase in the release of the endorphins and oxytocin hormones. When endorphins and oxytocin are released, your stress levels are reduced and you experience a deep sense of well-being, calm and contentment.

> **Yoga Parenting Tip:**
> Encourage your child to sit with you when you meditate. If they are not interested, don't force them; the more you practice, they will quickly pick up your calmer vibes and just by observing you, will notice the difference regular practice makes to your life.

So, how can you achieve calm and clarity during your chaotic and often confusing, life?

Seven Simple Steps to a Successful Meditation

Learning to meditate is a skill and a gift you give to yourself. If you are new to meditation, the following seven steps will give you a head start in setting up your own meditation practice.

- Find a quiet, comfortable space, in which you can sit undisturbed for a period of between 5-20 minutes.
- Find a sitting position that feels comfortable to you—maybe put a cushion on the floor and sit on it in a comfortable, cross-legged position. If your knees do not reach the floor or your hips feel stiff, let your knees rest on a couple of cushions. If it is more comfortable for you, sit on a straight back chair. If you sit on a chair, make sure your feet are flat on the ground, with your toes pointing forward.
- Make sure you sit up straight, and have your head, neck, and back aligned in a straight line. Rest your hands on your lap with the palms facing up.
- Close your eyes, take three deep breaths to clear your mind and prepare your mind for your practice.
- Close your eyes, and take a deep, steady breath—in through your nose—and as you breathe out, relax your shoulders and allow your jaw to relax.

- Take a slow, steady breath in, and then on the next exhale, allow your buttocks, thighs, calves, and feet to relax.
- Stay focused on your breathing. Breathe naturally, slowly, and gently, in and out through your nose. If your mind wanders and you lose your concentration, just return your awareness to your breathing. Keep your attention focused on your breath for at least five to ten cycles (inhale/exhale) of steady breathing.
- Gradually open your eyes. Stay seated for a few more moments to notice how you feel and to honor your intention to be calm, relaxed and maintain a gentler approach to life.

Yoga for Beginner's Tip:

Start off your mornings with two to ten minutes of meditation; you will feel calm, alert and, mentally prepared to respond in a peaceful, positive and proactive manner to events.

Case Study:

A former yoga student of mine, Ally, a 36-year-old accountant with a young baby, suffered from Lupus. Her medical treatments often left her feeling drained, exhausted, and struggling to care for her baby and manage work. Ally found meditation an ideal tool to help calm her nerves and help her relax and feel in control of her body during the intensive and sometimes invasive medical procedures.

What Ally Did When I Taught Her This Meditation
She would imagine herself inside a pink bubble, bathed in golden light. Once inside her bubble, and focusing on her breathing, she felt her spirit grow calm, no longer under attack, and she found peace with the demanding medical treatments.

Three Simple Meditation Techniques to Help You Let Go of Worries, Relax and Find Calm

Meditation Technique #1

Observe Your Breath

- Find a quiet space where you can sit undisturbed for 5-20 minutes.
- Sit in a comfortable position, either on the floor in suitable cross-legged position or on a chair.
- Make sure your spine is straight and if sitting on a chair rest your feet on the floor, legs uncrossed.
- Rest your hands in your lap, close your eyes and turn your attention to your breath.
- Spend a few moments observing your every -day breath and then slowly, allow your breath to soften and deepen as you simply focus on observing the rhythm of your breath, as you breath in and breathe out through your nose.
- If your mind wanders away from observing your breath, simple return your awareness to your breath and continue to focus on your breath.
- Continue with this practice for 5-20 minutes.
- Then slowly open your eyes, sit still for a few more moments, before re-engaging with your day.

Meditation Technique #2

Count Your Breath

- Sit in a comfortable position, either on the floor in suitable cross-legged position or on a chair.
- Make sure your spine is straight and if sitting on a chair rest your feet on the floor, legs uncrossed.
- Rest your hands in your lap, close your eyes and turn your attention to your breath.

- Become aware of your breath.
- Breathe in slowly through your nose and mentally count "one".
- Slowly breathe out and count "two".
- Breathe in and count "three", breathe out and count "four".
- Continue counting your in and out breath up to number 10.
- When you reach number 10, go back to number one and repeat the practice for 5-20 minutes.

If you mind wanders during the practice and you lose concentration, just return your attention to the breath and begin counting from number one.

Meditation Technique #3
Candle Meditation/Tratak Meditation

Sit on the floor or on a chair with a lighted candle in front of you. Gaze at the flame through half-closed eyes. Then close your eyes and visualise the warm glow from the candle behind your eyelids. Stay focused on this image. If you lose the image, gently open your eyes and gaze at the flame. Then close your eyes and repeat. Continue with this practice for 5 – 10 minutes. You can also practice tratak meditation outside in nature by focusing on a natural object, the moon or a bright star at night. With practice, you will quite easily be able to visualise your chosen object when you close your eyes.

When your meditations are completed, sit quietly for 2 minutes before engaging with your day.

5

FINAL THOUGHTS FOR A CALMER, HAPPIER YOU

ALL THE TIPS and suggestions in this book are activities my clients and I practice to help us reduce stress, relax and have energy to do the things which matter most to us.

I have shared these techniques here to inspire and encourage you to take time out of your daily schedule to take care of *you*.

I want you to feel relaxed, to know how to soothe away stress and find calm, especially when you have to juggle the demands of running a busy household, care for your family and keep on top of matters at work.

Here are three final thoughts I wish to share with you…

1 Stretch

Whenever you can, stretch your body. You can practice easy yoga poses at home or at work at your desk any time you feel your mind going into overdrive. Simple chair yoga exercises work wonders for relieving stress and re-energizing your body and mind. An easy, seated twist brings fresh oxygen and energy to your torso and massages your digestive organs.

2. Breathe Deeply

Yoga breathing exercises are the quickest way to slow down your thoughts, release anxiety and worry and calm your mind. Anytime you feel overwhelmed or aren't sure what to do next, sit down, and take a deep breath in through your nose and then slowly breathe out through your nose. Allow your shoulders to relax, and release tension in your jaw. Repeat this process for five to ten cycles of deep, steady breathing.

3. Spend Time Alone

Relax, and spend at least five to 15 minutes every day practicing meditation. Choose one of the techniques outlined in this book, and try it out for the next five days. I guarantee you will notice a difference in how you feel and respond to things.

Most importantly, be gentle, slow down, rest when you can, and enjoy each day of your life.

Namaste,

Ntathu Allen

Glossary of the Key Yoga Terms Used in This Book

Anuloma Viloma - The Sankrit term for the breathing exercise known as Alternate Nostril breathing.

Asana - Is the term used to describe a yoga posture, or yoga exercise.

Brahmari - Another name for the "Bumble Bee" breathing exercise.

Prana - Life energy, the life force.

Pranayama - The yogic term for breathing exercises, whereby you consciously regulate your breath

Tratak - A meditation technique used to aid concentration and focus - tratak is a 'steady gaze'.

Yoga - Means to yoke, union, to unite. Traditionally yoga is a system to help the individual soul unite with the Absolute.

Yogi (masculine), **Yogini** (feminine) - A person, who practices yoga.

ABOUT THE AUTHOR

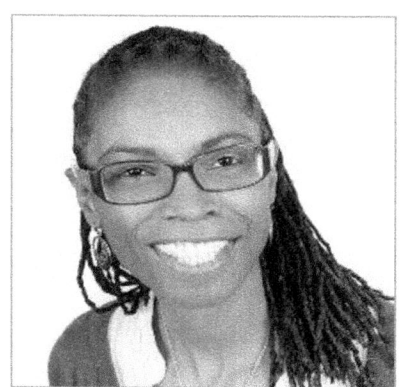

NTATHU IS A writer, yoga and meditation teacher who inspires and supports busy women to experience more pleasure and delight in their lives. She offers simple, self-care yoga exercises and techniques you can do at home or at work to help you release worry, feel calmer and more creative and focused. Mother of three imaginative, young-adult daughters, Ntathu uses yoga to remain joyful, balanced, and healthy. She offers free blog articles with weekly subscriptions via her website.

Visit: **www.yogainspires.co.uk** for your FREE guide to *Three Simple Strategies to Go from Crazy-Busy to Blissfully Calm – in as Little as Two Minutes.*

You Can Also Connect with Ntathu on…

Twitter: **twitter.com/yogainspiresyou**

Blog: **yogainspires.co.uk**

Facebook: **www.facebook.com/yogainspires**

LinkedIn: **www.linkedin.com/groups/Yoga-Inspires-Life-One-Breath-3702115**

OTHER BOOKS BY NTATHU

Yoga Basics For Beginners: A Simple Guide To Yoga For Beginners For Health, Fitness And Happiness (Yoga For Beginners Guide Book Book 2)

Work Happy!: 26 Quick And Easy Relaxation Tips To Help You Breeze Through Your Day

Healing After Loss: 28 Devotional Poems For Healing And Peace (Religion And Spirituality Books)

How To Love Yourself More: 365 Motivational Quotes & Affirmations To Kick-Start Your Day!

Back Care - Yoga Exercises For Lower Back Care At Work: Reduce Stress, Boost Energy And Improve Posture (Stress Management Techniques) (Back Pain Relief Treatment Book 1)

Mom And Me Have Fun Baking Thanksgiving Cupcakes (Thanksgiving Book For Children) (Children's Cookbooks For Holidays And Celebrations 1)

Do You Know If Kindle Unlimited Is For You?: The Ultimate Guide To The Benefits Of Kindle Unlimited For Avid Readers

Pray As You Go: Seven Meditation Techniques You Wish You Knew For Healing And Happiness (Guided Meditations For Beginners)

Yoga For Beginners: Your Complete Guide To Detox Your Body And Calm Your Mind (Yoga For Beginners Guide Books Book 1

Meditation For Beginners: The Essential Guide To Reduce Stress and Anxiety and Live A Healthy, Calm and Happy Life

Love Your Life!: 26 Inspirational Poems to Nurture Your Spirit through Hard Times (Spirituality & Personal Growth Book 1)

Visit Ntathu's Amazon Author Central Page—**http://www.amazon.com/Ntathu-Allen/e/B0085F6XAl** to find out more…

ACKNOWLEDGEMENTS

MANY PEOPLE HAVE kindly supported me through my journey…

My beautiful daughters, Hasina, Maleka, and Jameela, my parents, Victor and Cynthia Howell, my brother John and Cousin Sherry, whose passing led me to discover yoga. Shola Arewa, my yoga teacher, for introducing me to the gift of yoga; Judy Cullins, my book coach, for her intuitive eye and humorous book-coaching sessions, and Peter Woodhead, who introduced me to the infinite possibilities of internet marketing as a tool for sharing the gifts of yoga. Special thanks to Jamie Whipham for bringing my words to life with his magical illustrations.

May you be blessed with a graceful body, peace of mind, and a grateful heart.

Your Free Gift

AS A WAY of saying thanks for your purchase, I'm offering a free video that is exclusive to my book and blog readers.

In *Soothe Away Stress*, you'll discover 3 simple ways you can use to quickly go from crazy-busy to blissfully calm in just 2 minutes. You can easily fit these 3 simple techniques into your busy schedule, and do them anywhere, anytime, you feel overwhelmed, distracted and anxious and need to relax, focus and be calm.

Go to the following URL to get your free Soothe Away Stress video

http://yogainspires.co.uk

GET SPECIAL DEALS ON MORE BEST SELLING BOOKS

Get discounts and special deals on our best selling books at
www.tckpublishing.com/bookdeals

Index

A

affirmations 33
alcoholism 3
American Medical Association 4
anxiety 3, 4, 46, 52, 68
asanas .... *See* Yoga Poses

B

back pain 25
blood pressure 5
Breath:
    anger 43
    deep breathing exercise 46
    exercise for posture 48
    mind-body connection 43
    work exercise 47
Breathing Exercises:
    Alternate Nostril Breathing
        (Anuloma Viloma) 56–58
    beat stress & restore energy 51
    Bumble Bee breath 54
    Single Nostril Breathing 55

C

Case Studies:
    stiff hips 33
    back pain 25
    emotional relief 29
    meditation 59, 64
    seniors 50
    stress 9–10
chronic illness 2

computer use 14
Concentration:
    and meditation 69
    as benefit of yoga 52
    difficulty 4
    loss 64

D

depression 3
divorce 6, 29, 44
drug dependency 3

E

endorphins 62
energy 6, 11, 45, 69

F

family yoga time 36
fatigue 5, 64
flexibility 6, 24, 28
focus 7, 44, 51, 58, 69

G

glossary 69

H

hormones 62

L

Lupus 64

M

massage 27, 28, 39
Meditation:
    benefits 61–62
    steps to success 63
Meditation Techniques:
    Candle Meditation aka Tratak
        Meditation 66
    counting the breath 65–66
    observing the breath 65
menstruation 33
morning stretches 12

O

overwork 3
oxygen 13, 42, 68

P

Parenting Tips .27, 28, 31, 35, 37, 44, 48, 53, 54, 63
peace 13, 43, 59, 61, 62, 64
pregnancy 33
pulse rate 5

R

rest 3, 39, 43

S

shoulders, rounded 49
sleeping problems 38
Soothe Away Stress [video] 77
stiffness 14, 24, 25, 30
Stress:
    chronic illness 2
    killer 4
    relief through yoga 6
    signs 4–5
    work/overwork 3
    workplace 3
stress-free fact 2

stress-free yoga tip 5
stretches for stiffness & pain 14

T

thought energy 47
time management 62
Tratak Meditation 66

W

worry 5, 6, 7, 10, 41, 68

Y

Yoga for Beginner's Tips:
    beginning 14
    breathing 12, 13, 43, 44, 48, 56
    breathing breaks 45
    emotional relief 47, 51
    gentleness 23
    inflexibility 34
    mornings 64
    positioning 25, 27, 30, 32, 52
    posture 37
    power of the breath 42
    relaxation 39
    vitality 53
Yoga Poses:
    arms above head 17
    backward bend 20
    child's pose 31
    cobbler pose 33
    cobra 28
    feet & ankle stretch 15
    knee to chest/spinal massage 24
    lean on me 36
    neck stretch 16
    seated forward bend 19, 26
    seated rag doll 39
    spinal twist 22
    straight arms behind back 49
    stretches for stiffness & pain 14
    trunk twist 21

www.ingramcontent.com/pod-product-compliance
Lightning Source LLC
Chambersburg PA
CBHW071117030426
42336CB00013BA/2121